Rhabdomyolysis

The Ultimate Guide to Empower Your Health

Palrmer O. Stocker

DISCLAIMER

Table of Contents

Introduction

✓ Understanding Rhabdomyolysis

Comprehending Rhabdomyolysis: Taking Charge of Your Own Muscle Health

Imagine your muscles abruptly turning against you—tiny powerhouses that have been working nonstop to propel your movement. The dangerous disorder known as rhabdomyolysis, or "rhabdo," is caused by the breakdown of those powerhouses, which releases noxious compounds into your bloodstream. Although it may sound frightening, knowing about rhabdo gives you the ability to safeguard your health and use it wisely.

Dissecting the Fundamentals:

"What is it?" Rhabdo is a condition when injured muscle tissue leaks its contents into the bloodstream, which includes the dangerous protein myoglobin. Your kidneys may be strained as a result, which could have major consequences.

• "What is the cause?" Severe heatstroke and intense activity in hot weather are the usual culprits. On the other hand, drugs, infections, genetics, and even pharmaceutical addiction can cause rhabdo.

• "What signs are present?" Important symptoms include disorientation, black urine, weakness, and muscle discomfort. Intervention and early detection are essential.

<u>Building Your Own Power</u>:

• Knowledge is power. Being aware of the various reasons and risk factors enables you to make well-informed decisions regarding your lifestyle, prescription drugs, and general health.

• Prevention is key: Avoid overheating, stay hydrated, and pay attention to your body when exercising. Know the possible adverse effects of your medications and talk to your doctor about them.

• Early identification is essential. Learn about the symptoms and get help right away if you think you may have rhabdo.

• Genetic predisposition: Although uncommon, certain people are predisposed to rhabdo due to genetics. It can be beneficial to discuss this with your doctor and be aware of your family history.
• Recovery and Beyond: If you have gone through rhabdo, you can take charge of your path by learning about the recovery process, handling any long-term repercussions, and getting in touch with support groups.
• Advocacy and research: You can help advance the prevention, diagnosis, and treatment of rhabdo by spreading the word about this condition and funding research projects.

You can protect your muscular health and effectively manage rhabdo by arming yourself with knowledge and taking proactive measures. Recall that you are not traveling alone!

Chapter 1: Muscle Mayhem Unveiled: What is Rhabdomyolysis and Why Should You Care?

Rapid skeletal muscle disintegration that releases intracellular muscle components into the bloodstream and extracellular space is known as rhabdomyolysis, a dangerous medical disorder. Numerous circumstances, such as trauma, immobility, sepsis, cardiovascular operations, overexertion, heat exposure, and some drugs or poisonous chemicals, might contribute to this condition.

Acute renal injury, electrolyte imbalances, and disseminated intravascular coagulation are among the systemic consequences that can arise from the release of muscle components, such as myoglobin, creatine kinase, and electrolytes.

Rhabdomyolysis can cause muscle weakness, discomfort, swelling, and dark red urine from myoglobinuria, among other clinical symptoms. Early diagnosis and therapy are critical for a successful recovery from rhabdomyolysis, and prompt detection of the condition is critical to avert any complications.

Workers in a variety of occupations are more vulnerable to rhabdomyolysis because it is linked to heat exposure, physical effort, misuse, and direct damage in the workplace.

Supportive therapies for rhabdomyolysis usually include maintaining renal function and correcting electrolyte abnormalities. To avoid major medical issues and long-term detrimental health impacts, early action is essential.

Healthcare providers and patients alike must have a thorough understanding of the origins, symptoms, and management of rhabdomyolysis because patients' prognoses can be greatly impacted by prompt diagnosis and effective therapy.

Chapter 2: Beyond the Usual Suspects: Unveiling the Diverse Causes of Rhabdo

Above and Beyond the Sweat and Heat: Exposing the Surprising Causes of Rhabdomyolysis

Rhabdomyolysis, or "rhabdo," is commonly associated with heatstroke or intense activity. Even though there are typical triggers, there are unexpectedly many other interesting players in this muscular meltdown than the typical suspects. Let's learn more about the less well-known causes of rhabdo to empower ourselves:

1. The Men in the Medicine Cabinet:

• Statins: Although generally safe, these cholesterol-lowering medications rarely cause rhabdo, especially when taken in combination with other medications or during vigorous physical activity.

• Antipsychotics: In hot temperatures or when dehydrated, some mental drugs, especially those from older groups like phenothiazines, can cause rhabdo.

• Antibiotics: Due to their potential to interfere with muscle metabolism, certain antibiotics, such as macrolides and fluoroquinolones, have been connected to rhabdo.

• Recreational Drugs: By directly harming muscle tissue or raising body temperature, cocaine, ecstasy, and even amphetamines can result in rhabdo.

2. Contagious Enemies:

• Viral Infections: Rarely, rhabdo can be brought on by influenza, dengue fever, or even a regular cold. This is probably because of the body's inflammatory reaction.
• Parasitic Infections: Parasites like toxoplasmosis and trichinosis can invade muscle tissue and cause rhabdo, which is frequently accompanied by muscle pain and weakness. Severe bacterial infections, such as sepsis, can also cause rhabdo due to widespread inflammation and tissue damage.

3. The Twist in the Genetic Predisposition Plot:

• Malignant Hyperthermia Susceptibility: This hereditary disorder can cause some anesthetic medications used during surgery to cause a potentially fatal rhabdo-like reaction.
• Carnitine Deficiency Disorders: Rhabdomyolysis can occur with exercise or effort due to some hereditary disorders that impact muscle energy metabolism.
• Other Genetic Mutations: Studies are beginning to identify connections between certain gene mutations and a heightened vulnerability to rhabdo in some scenarios.

Through comprehension of these several reasons, we can take an active role in maintaining our health:

• Be knowledgeable about medications. Consult your doctor about possible interactions and side effects, particularly if you have risk factors.
Practice informed drug use: Pay close attention to dosage instructions, and don't be afraid to ask questions.

• Be on the lookout for infections: Discuss any odd symptoms, such as muscle soreness, with your doctor and seek immediate medical assistance for serious infections.

• Be aware of your family history: See your doctor about genetic testing or special precautions if there is a family history of rhabdo or related diseases.

Keep in mind: This information should not be used in place of expert medical advice; rather, it is intended solely for educational reasons. Always seek the advice and diagnosis of your physician.

• Spread the word about the various causes of rhabdo to family and friends. Push for more money and research to advance our knowledge of and ability to treat this difficult condition.

• Encourage groups whose mission is to empower and educate rhabdo victims.
We may empower ourselves for a healthier future by protecting ourselves and others from the unanticipated causes of rhabdo by remaining aware and adopting proactive measures.

Chapter 3: From Aches to Alarms: Recognizing the Signs and Symptoms of Rhabdo

Rhabdomyolysis: Recognizing the Indications and Manifestations

Rapid skeletal muscle destruction and subsequent release of intracellular muscle components into the circulation and extracellular space are hallmarks of the dangerous medical disorder known as rhabdomyolysis. This disorder is linked to a number of symptoms and complications, some of which are potentially fatal.

Rhabdomyolysis Common Symptoms: Weakness, stiffness, and pain in the muscles, dark urine, (which myoglobinuria can cause to appear red or brown). Muscle swelling, Exhaustion or weakness, Vomiting and nausea

Additional Indications and Signs

- Blood levels of creatine kinase (CK) may rise sharply.
- Unexpectedly acute aches, pains, or cramps in the muscles.
- Dehydration.
- Exposure to heat.
- Usage of illegal drugs or certain medications.

Direct trauma: One of the conditions known as rhabdomyolysis, which is characterized by the disintegration of muscle fibers, is direct trauma. Both blunt and crush injuries have the potential to cause trauma-induced rhabdomyolysis. Infections, medications, toxins, metabolic and electrolyte imbalances, genetic abnormalities, and medicines are additional risk factors for rhabdomyolysis. Rhabdomyolysis manifests clinically as muscle soreness, weakness, dark tea-colored urine, and a noticeable increase in serum creatine kinase levels. Continuous evaluation of breathing, circulation, and airway; proper hydration; close monitoring of urine output; correction of electrolyte abnormalities; and detection of complications such as compartment syndrome and disseminated intravascular coagulation are all part of the management of rhabdomyolysis. Steer clear of strenuous physical activity, be properly hydrated, and take care of any underlying medical issues in order to prevent rhabdomyolysis.

Heat exposure: Rhabdomyolysis is a dangerous medical illness that can be fatal or leave a person permanently disabled. Heat exposure is a risk factor for this ailment. Rhabdomyolysis can occur in the workplace as a result of heat exposure, physical strain or overuse, and direct trauma (such as a fall-related crush injury).

Rhabdomyolysis is more common in workers in a wide range of occupations, including sports, police officers, firefighters, first responders, and those in agriculture and construction. It is imperative to stay hydrated, take pauses in a cooler location, recognize the warning signals of heat-related illnesses, and avoid jobs or recreational activities that require exertion and/or heat exposure if at all feasible in order to prevent rhabdomyolysis. By enforcing heat stress management procedures, permitting and encouraging workers to seek medical attention when experiencing signs of rhabdomyolysis, and pushing workers to use sick days when they're ill, employers can help prevent their workers from acquiring rhabdomyolysis.

Immobility: Serious side effects of rhabdomyolysis include muscle damage and the bloodstream's release of intracellular components. Acute kidney injury (AKI) and renal failure are among the consequences that can arise from this condition. One of the risk factors for rhabdomyolysis is immobility, especially after stressful events that limit mobility or during extended bed rest.

Rhabdomyolysis linked to immobility is at risk for:

1. Extended bed rest following surgery or an injury.
2. Compartment syndrome, which can appear in immobile patients following fluid resuscitation.

3. Third-degree burns, lightning strikes, or electrical shock injuries that can become immobile.

Prevention methods for rhabdomyolysis associated with immobility:

1. Prompt mobilization and recuperation following surgery or injury
2. Frequently shifting the patient's posture to encourage blood flow and avoid pressure sores
3. Keeping an eye out for compartment syndrome symptoms and acting quickly to treat them
4. Promoting exercise and physical activity within the patient's limits
5. Making sure you have enough food and water to maintain the health of your muscles

In cases of rhabdomyolysis, early identification and treatment are essential for reducing complications and improving outcomes.
Important therapeutic approaches consist of:

1. Using normal saline and isotonic fluids for aggressive fluid resuscitation in order to keep the urine output target of 200 mL/hour.
2. To reduce muscle injury, the offending agent must be located and removed.

3. Keeping an eye on and treating side effects includes compartment syndrome, acute renal damage, and electrolyte imbalances.

To sum up, rhabdomyolysis can be caused by immobility, and early mobilization, frequent position changes, and problem monitoring are effective preventive measures. Timely diagnosis and treatment are crucial to reducing problems and enhancing results.

Sepsis: Rhabdomyolysis Seizures: Risk Factors and Prevention

One of the main causes of morbidity and death in rhabdomyolysis patients is sepsis. Numerous case reports and original research investigations have established a link between rhabdomyolysis and sepsis.

Rhabdomyolysis caused by sepsis is susceptible to:

1. The most common causes of sepsis-induced rhabdomyolysis are thought to be gram-positive bacterial infections, such as Streptococcus species and Staphylococcus aureus.
2. Rhabdomyolysis is also linked to gram-negative bacterial infections such as Escherichia coli, Klebsiella, and pseudomonas.

3. Sepsis in rhabdomyolysis frequently centers on lung infections.

Prevention methods for rhabdomyolysis brought on by sepsis:

1. Early detection and management of sepsis, encompassing suitable antibiotic treatment and source control measures.
2. Avoiding nosocomial infections by closely adhering to infection control protocols.
3. Prompt identification and treatment of rhabdomyolysis risk factors, including persistent drinking, statin use, hypokalemia, hypernatremia, and hypophosphatemia.

Prompt diagnosis and treatment of rhabdomyolysis caused by sepsis are essential for reducing complications and enhancing results. Important therapeutic approaches consist of:

1. To maintain a urine output goal of 200 mL/hour, aggressive fluid resuscitation with isotonic fluids and normal saline is recommended.
2. To reduce the risk of more muscle damage, the offending chemical must be located and removed.

3. Keeping an eye on and treating side effects such as compartment syndrome, acute renal damage, and electrolyte imbalances.

In summary, gram-positive and gram-negative bacterial infections are the most common causes of rhabdomyolysis, and sepsis is a significant contributing factor. Prompt sepsis identification and treatment, together with the control of rhabdomyolysis risk factors, are preventative measures. Reducing problems and enhancing results require early detection and intervention.

Cardiovascular surgery: A disorder known as rhabdomyolysis is characterized by the quick disintegration of injured skeletal muscle, which releases intracellular muscle components into the blood. One of the causes of rhabdomyolysis is cardiovascular surgery, which is linked to particular risk factors and consequences.

'Risk Elements and Results':
According to a study, 19% of patients had rhabdomyolysis following heart surgery. Longer operation times, longer pump times, intraoperative hemodynamic instability, and prior statin use were risk factors for rhabdomyolysis following heart surgery.

Although rhabdomyolysis after heart surgery is common in patients with a history of statin usage or intraoperative hemodynamic instability, it has little bearing on the midterm prognosis.

Higher serum myoglobin levels following heart surgery and excess weight in obese patients are associated with higher mortality and the requirement for renal replacement therapy.

Management and Prevention:

Early monitoring, sufficient padding for appropriate placement, cutting down on operating time, sufficient hydration, and careful postoperative monitoring are all important in the prevention and management of rhabdomyolysis after heart surgery.

Depending on the severity and etiology of rhabdomyolysis, patients who experience it after cardiac surgery may need to be admitted to the intensive care unit and consult with critical care, nephrology, trauma surgery, vascular surgery, or orthopedic surgery.

In conclusion, rhabdomyolysis is a recognized side effect after heart surgery, and some risk factors have been found, including the use of statins and intraoperative hemodynamic instability. For the therapy of rhabdomyolysis in this setting, early monitoring and preventive measures—like sufficient padding for appropriate posture and close postoperative monitoring—are crucial.

Overuse: A complicated medical disorder known as rhabdomyolysis causes injured skeletal muscle to dissolve quickly, releasing intracellular muscle components into the bloodstream. Rhabdomyolysis is known to be caused by overuse of muscles, which can be brought on by narcotics, alcohol, cocaine, amphetamines, and other substances, as well as by exercising to an extreme degree, especially in persons who are not trained. Rhabdomyolysis is also frequently caused by trauma, immobilization, and heat-related injuries.

Rhabdomyolysis can present with a wide range of clinical symptoms, from asymptomatic to frequently associated with symptoms such as abrupt muscle weakness, pain, soreness, and edema in the affected extremity or body part. Urine that has darkened (tea-colored) may also be prevalent. Early detection of rhabdomyolysis is essential to avoiding difficulties later on. Urine dipstick testing is one kind of screening that can be used.

In order to improve end-organ perfusion, the management of rhabdomyolysis should involve regular examinations, close monitoring of urine output, correction of electrolyte abnormalities, ongoing assessment of breathing, circulation, and airway, as well as identification of complications such as compartment syndrome and disseminated intravascular coagulation.

In summary, rhabdomyolysis can result from overusing muscles, particularly when doing so during an unfamiliar or intense physical activity. For those who are at risk of developing problems and for their outcomes to be improved, early detection and treatment are crucial.
Overdoing it: Going Overboard in Rhabdomyolysis Risk Assessment and Management

A serious muscle injury that results in the release of intracellular muscle components into the bloodstream is known as rhabdomyolysis. Excessive physical exercise, particularly when combined with intense effort, can result in rhabdomyolysis. Important risk factors and techniques for preventing overindulgence in it include:

'Perilous Elements':
Excessive physical effort; dehydration; overuse of muscles, particularly during resistance training; and usage of drugs or substances known to induce muscular injury, including cocaine, alcohol, amphetamines, and some pharmaceuticals.

'Preventive Techniques':
- Seek advice from an exercise professional before beginning resistance training; - Start with training loads of 60–70% for 8 to 12 repetitions, and don't do more than 1 to 3 sets per exercise when starting out; - Stay well-hydrated before, during, and after physical activity; - Avoid excessive use of drugs or substances that can cause muscle damage; - Gradually increase the intensity and duration of physical activity to avoid overuse.

For those who are at risk of rhabdomyolysis, early diagnosis and treatment are essential to avoiding complications and achieving better results. Preventing acute kidney injury, addressing electrolyte imbalances, and controlling side effects such as compartment syndrome and disseminated intravascular coagulation are important therapy objectives.

Intense exercise without a break: Preventing Rhabdomyolysis from Intense Exercise and Risk Factors

A disorder called rhabdomyolysis, which is defined as the disintegration of muscle fibers, can arise from strenuous exercise, particularly when people push themselves beyond their comfort zones. The main risk factors and mitigation techniques for rhabdomyolysis brought on by vigorous exercise are as follows:

Intensity of Exercise: Sudden, vigorous physical activity, especially above one's normal limitations, might result in rhabdomyolysis. Here are some risk factors for the condition:

Dehydration: Inadequate fluid consumption before, during, and after physical activity raises the possibility of rhabdomyolysis.

Environmental Factors: Rhabdomyolysis risk may increase with hot and muggy exercise conditions.

Substance Use: Taking large amounts of creatine-containing supplements or highly caffeinated energy drinks prior to exercise may increase your chance of developing rhabdomyolysis.

Prevention Strategies:
Gradual Progression: To reduce the risk of rhabdomyolysis, people should gradually introduce new or vigorous exercise regimens, especially after a period of inactivity.

Hydration: To avoid dehydration and lower the risk of rhabdomyolysis, it is essential to consume enough fluids before, during, and after exercise.

Awareness of Limits: When exercising, it's critical to understand and respect one's physical limitations. To avoid overexertion, people should slow down or stop if they are having difficulty.

Medical Consultation: People should see a healthcare provider to make sure they are healthy enough before beginning a new fitness regimen, particularly if it involves vigorous exercise.

For people who may have overexerted themselves and are exhibiting symptoms that might point to rhabdomyolysis, early diagnosis and treatment are crucial. People should seek medical assistance as soon as they feel concerned in order to avoid problems related to this potentially dangerous condition.

In summary, environmental variables, dehydration, and vigorous exercise are linked to the risk of rhabdomyolysis. People can lessen their chance of having rhabdomyolysis by gradually increasing the intensity of their exercise, drinking plenty of water, being conscious of their own limitations, and consulting a doctor.

Specific genetic disorders: Certain genetic abnormalities can induce rhabdomyolysis, but because of their relative rarity and great variety, diagnosing them can be difficult. After a thorough evaluation of all rhabdomyolysis patients across the hospital, with an emphasis on genetic and environmental causes, pathogenic variations in 22 distinct genes were discovered. These variants are expected to enhance the vulnerability to rhabdomyolysis. Furthermore, the broad genetic spectrum underlying rhabdomyolysis susceptibility is expanded by the probable involvement of 11 genes in enhanced susceptibility. For each gene, the clinical phenotype, common causes of rhabdomyolysis, and suggested diagnostic strategy have been examined. Depending on the age at which the condition manifests, a number of factors can cause rhabdomyolysis from genetic abnormalities, including mental stress, extended aerobic exercise, fasting, cold weather, shivering, and other catabolic stressors, including fever and infections. Examining the patient's symptoms in connection to the type and timing of exercise, blood creatinine levels, inheritance pattern, and rhabdomyolysis triggers is part of the diagnostic process.

Dehydration: Rhabdomyolysis does not directly cause dehydration, but it can exacerbate the illness. A muscle injury results in rhabdomyolysis, which allows the body to absorb proteins and electrolytes. Organ damage may result from dehydration's detrimental effects on the body's capacity to eliminate electrolytes and muscle proteins. Additionally, dehydration can decrease blood flow to the kidneys, raising the possibility of renal injury. As a result, in order to avoid dehydration and lower the chance of rhabdomyolysis, it's critical to maintain adequate hydration before, during, and after physical activity. In addition, maintaining enough hydration is essential for managing rhabdomyolysis because it enhances end-organ perfusion and guards against acute renal failure. Early identification and treatment are crucial for minimizing complications and improving outcomes in persons at risk of rhabdomyolysis, in addition to maintaining enough hydration.

Usage of illegal drugs or certain medications:
Certain medications or the use of illegal narcotics might cause rhabdomyolysis. According to a Euro-DEN study, the most frequent substances that cause rhabdomyolysis include heroin, cocaine, amphetamine, cannabis, GHB/GBL, and amphetamine. These drugs can cause rhabdomyolysis via a number of different routes, including direct toxicity and overuse of the muscles. Moreover, myotoxic medications or intravenous drug usage can directly cause muscle damage, and prolonged seizures or insufficient blood flow can create secondary muscular injuries that can lead to drug-induced rhabdomyolysis. The seriousness of acute rhabdomyolysis is highlighted by the estimated 5% to 25% of cases that result in renal failure due to

drug-induced causes. Therefore, the risk of rhabdomyolysis and its related problems, such as kidney damage and failure, can be greatly increased by using illegal drugs or specific prescriptions. People should seek medical assistance if they have symptoms of rhabdomyolysis after using these substances and be aware of the possible risks associated with them.

Care and Handling

Supportive treatment, which includes correcting electrolyte imbalances and maintaining renal function.
Prompt action is essential to avoid major medical issues and long-term detrimental health effects

Multidisciplinary Approach:

Consulting with experts in several fields, including nutrition, endocrinology, cardiology, nephrologists, and internists, guarantees that your recuperation takes into account every aspect of your health.

Prevention: Adopt a healthy lifestyle, abstain from excessive alcohol and drug usage, and stay hydrated.
Take precautions to ensure that rhabdomyolysis doesn't occur again if it has.

Get medical help right away if you think you could have rhabdomyolysis. A complete recovery depends on early diagnosis and treatment.

Chapter 4: A Diagnostic Deep Dive: How Doctors Identify and Confirm Rhabdo

In order to avoid major problems, rhabdomyolysis is a difficult medical disorder that needs to be diagnosed and treated right away. A mix of imaging investigations, laboratory testing, and clinical characteristics are used to diagnose rhabdomyolysis. Muscle soreness, weakness, and black urine from myoglobinuria make up the traditional triad of symptoms. Less than 10% of patients exhibit this trio; hence, further helpful hints might include the presence of muscular damage accompanied by an unanticipated increase in serum phosphate or aspartate aminotransferase levels.

Serum creatine kinase (CK) level detection is the most sensitive laboratory test for rhabdomyolysis diagnosis. The most accurate test for rhabdomyolysis brought on by muscular damage is elevated CK levels. However, there may be a mismatch between the degree of muscle damage and the likelihood of difficulties when it comes to CK levels. Myoglobin, lactate dehydrogenase, and electrolyte levels are additional laboratory tests that could be helpful in the diagnosis of rhabdomyolysis.

The diagnosis of rhabdomyolysis may also benefit from imaging tests including computed tomography (CT), magnetic resonance imaging (MRI), and ultrasonography. The underlying cause and degree of muscle damage can be revealed by these imaging tests, and the affected muscles usually show hypertrophy, edema, and hemorrhage.

Early diagnosis and therapy are necessary for a full recovery from rhabdomyolysis, and prompt detection of the condition is crucial to preventing late complications. Get medical help right away if you think you could have rhabdomyolysis.

✓ Taking Control: Preventing and Managing Rhabdo

A Complete Guide to Avoiding and Treating Rhabdo

When working in the heat, stay hydrated and steer clear of low-sugar and caffeine-containing products.

Steer clear of alcohol when working in hot conditions.

- To avoid heat-related illnesses, take pauses in a cooler location.

- Before working for extended periods of time, acclimate yourself to physical activity and heat.

- Remain at home from work while ill because rhabdo is more common in various illnesses.

- Increase physical activity levels gradually, particularly when beginning a new workout regimen.

- Before beginning a new fitness regimen, speak with a doctor or fitness instructor.

- Steer clear of strenuous exercise, particularly if you have a history of rhabdo or other disorders affecting the muscles.

- Continue eating a lot of carbohydrates, particularly when you get acute presentations.

- Drink plenty of water, particularly when giving an acute presentation.

- Steer clear of intense exercise, particularly if you have long-chain fatty acid oxidation disorders (LC-FAOD).

Practice Safety

- Sip lots of water prior to, during, and following physical activity.
- Steer clear of anti-inflammatory drugs such as naproxen and ibuprofen.
- Steer clear of alcohol.
- Increase the length and intensity of exercise gradually.
- Throughout return-to-play programs, keep an eye on laboratory results and symptoms.

Progressive Increase in Exercise

- Begin with stretching, body-weight resistance exercises, core training, stationary cycling, and resistance training with elastic bands.
- Increase activity level as tolerated while keeping a close eye on lab results and symptoms.

Identifying Danger Signals

Myoglobinuria-related muscle soreness, weakness, and black urine.

Abdominal pain, nausea, vomiting, fever, a fast heartbeat, disorientation, dehydration, and unconsciousness are some more symptoms.

Getting Medical Help

- If you feel like you could have rhabdo, stop what you're doing, cool down, drink some water, and visit a doctor to have it checked out.
- Increasing fluid intake is the mainstay of home treatment for most cases of rhabdo.
- IV fluids may be required if there are indications of renal issues or if muscle enzyme levels are elevated.

Multidisciplinary Method

See experts like cardiologists, internists, nephrologists, endocrinologists, and nutritionists to make sure that every aspect of your recuperation is covered.

Endorsing a Comeback to Perform

Create a safe and efficient approach for returning to play based on the advice already in place, which should include instructions for ongoing laboratory and clinical monitoring.

You can greatly lower your chance of developing rhabdomyolysis and enhance your general health and wellbeing by adhering to these recommendations.

Chapter 5: Sweat Smart, Not Scary: Exercise Safety Tips to Avoid Rhabdo

In order to avoid rhabdomyolysis and ensure safe activity, implement the following 12 tips into your fitness regimen:

1. Remain Hydrated: To avoid dehydration, which can aggravate rhabdomyolysis, drink lots of water prior to, during, and after exercise.

2. Steadily Increase Intensity: Steer clear of abrupt, strenuous exercise. To give your body time to adjust, gradually boost the intensity and length of your workout.

3. Identify Danger Signals: Be alert for signs of rhabdomyolysis, such as intense muscle soreness, weakness, and dark urine. Abdominal pain, nausea, vomiting, fever, and a fast heartbeat are further symptoms.

4. Consult a healthcare professional: Speak with a fitness trainer or healthcare professional prior to beginning a new fitness program, particularly if you are inexperienced with exercise or have a history of medical issues.

5. Avoid Overexertion: Refrain from exerting yourself until you are in excruciating pain or weariness. Pay attention to your body and take pauses when required.

6. Eat a Balanced Diet: To sustain your energy levels while exercising, have a balanced diet that includes enough carbohydrates.

7. Avoid Alcohol and Caffeine: Since these substances can exacerbate dehydration and muscular soreness, avoid taking them either before or after exercise.

8. Use Proper Form: To avoid straining your muscles or injuring them, make sure you are performing your exercises with the proper form and technique.

9. Recovery and Rest: Give your body enough time to recuperate and rest in between sessions. Rhabdomyolysis risk might be raised by overtraining.

10. Monitor Symptoms: Get help right away if you have any strange or severe symptoms during or after activity, such as ongoing muscle soreness.

11. Warm-Up and Cool-Down: To prime your muscles for activity and speed up recovery, begin your workout with a good warm-up and finish with a cool-down.

12. Listen to Your Body: Be aware of the cues that your body gives you. If you feel sick or notice worrying symptoms, change your exercise regimen or contact a doctor.

You may lessen the chance of rhabdomyolysis and encourage a safe and efficient workout habit by implementing these exercise safety measures into your fitness practice.

Chapter 6: Medication Savvy: Understanding the Rhabdo Risks of Common Drugs

One rare but dangerous complication that can be brought on by many medications is rhabdomyolysis. Certain medications have the potential to directly damage muscles, while others can lead to dangerously high levels of physical activity, ischemia from constricted arteries, convulsions, or hyperthermia. Many regular pharmaceuticals and illicit drugs are included in the long list of drugs that might cause rhabdomyolysis. The following medications have been linked to rhabdomyolysis:

Statins: HMG-CoA reductase inhibitors, which are frequently used to reduce cholesterol, carry a higher risk of producing adverse effects in the skeletal muscle, either on their own or in conjunction with other medications.

Antipsychotics and antidepressants: Prolonged immobilization brought on by pressure-induced ischemia can result in rhabdomyolysis.

Sedative hypnotics: Rhabdomyolysis can be brought on by benzodiazepines, flunitrazepam, and nitrazepam.

Recreational drugs: Rhabdomyolysis has been linked to the use of cocaine, cannabis, GHB/GBL, amphetamine, and heroin.

Additional drugs: Rhabdomyolysis has also been linked to oxalactam, opioids, oxprenolol, paracetamol, penicillamine, pentamidine, phencyclidine, phenylpropanolamine, quinidine, salicylates, strychnine, theophylline, terbutaline, and thiazides.

Remember that this is not a complete list and that rhabdomyolysis can also be brought on by other medications. Seek immediate medical attention if you have symptoms like severe muscle pain, weakness, or black urine while taking any medicine. Before beginning any new drug or supplement, it's crucial to speak with a doctor or pharmacist to learn about the possible dangers and adverse effects.

Chapter 7: When Infections Turn Dangerous: Protecting Yourself from Rhabdo During Illness

Rapid skeletal muscle disintegration that releases intracellular muscle components into the bloodstream and extracellular space is known as rhabdomyolysis, a dangerous medical disorder. Although direct trauma is the most common cause, other causes include infections, muscle ischemia, metabolic and electrolyte imbalances, genetic disorders, physical exertion, extended bed rest, and temperature-induced conditions like neuroleptic malignant syndrome and malignant hyperthermia. The onset of rhabdomyolysis has been linked to bacterial and viral infections. Rhabdomyolysis has been linked to viral and bacterial illnesses, such as those brought on by the influenza A and B viruses and Legionella bacteria. Myalgia, weakness, and myoglobinuria are among the clinical signs of rhabdomyolysis. The most sensitive test for rhabdomyolysis caused by muscle injury is an increase in creatine kinase (CK) levels. It's critical to identify the telltale signs and symptoms of rhabdomyolysis, which include pain, stiffness, weakness, and changes in urine color, and to get medical help as soon as possible if these symptoms occur. It is important to be aware that rhabdomyolysis can occur as a complication in the context of infections and to keep an eye out for the distinctive signs, particularly in cases of severe illness. To avoid major consequences and encourage recovery, early diagnosis and treatment are crucial.

Chapter 8: Know Your Body, Know Your Risk: Genetic Predispositions and Rhabdo Awareness

Knowing the possible genetic factors that may raise the chance of getting rhabdomyolysis is crucial when thinking about genetic predispositions and rhabdomyolysis awareness. Educating people about the illness, its signs, and the value of genetic testing can also give them the power to make well-informed decisions about their health. Here are some essential details to incorporate within the text:

Hereditary Propensities for Rhabdomyolysis

1. Genetic Disorders: Talk about particular genetic disorders, such as muscular dystrophies, metabolic myopathies, and genetic faults influencing muscle metabolism, that may make a person more susceptible to rhabdomyolysis.

2. Inherited enzyme impairments Describe how rhabdomyolysis can be more likely in individuals with inherited impairments in muscle metabolism-related enzymes, such as myophosphorylase or carnitine palmitoyltransferase.

3. Pharmacogenetics: Examine how pharmacogenetics relates to rhabdomyolysis, specifically how genetic differences can affect a person's reaction to drugs that are known to raise the risk of the illness, including muscle relaxants and statins.

Genetic Testing and Awareness of Rhabdomyolysis

1. Symptom Recognition: Inform people about the warning signs and symptoms of rhabdomyolysis, such as black urine, weakness, and discomfort in the muscles, and stress the need to get medical help if these symptoms appear.

2. Family History: To determine their risk, people with a family history of rhabdomyolysis or similar genetic disorders should think about genetic counseling and testing.

3. Medication Management: Emphasize the need to talk to medical professionals about hereditary susceptibilities to rhabdomyolysis when taking drugs that are known to possibly aggravate the illness.

4. Lifestyle Considerations: To reduce the risk of rhabdomyolysis in those with genetic predispositions, emphasize the importance of genetic awareness when

making lifestyle decisions, such as food and exercise routines.

By giving people this knowledge, they can better comprehend the hereditary components of rhabdomyolysis and the value of genetic testing and proactive awareness in maintaining their health.

Chapter 9: Battling Back: Treatment Options and Management Strategies for Rhabdo

Rhabdomyolysis Treatment and Management Techniques

Treatment for rhabdomyolysis varies based on how severe the problem is. Less serious situations can be handled using:

Hydrating, Recuperating, and Steering clear of the heat

Severe to moderate instances might need:

Intravenous (IV) fluids to remove electrolytes and muscle proteins; hospital stay to monitor and manage any issues

Among the ways to manage difficulties are:

Cardiac monitoring, electrolyte imbalance, and irregular heartbeat medication
Physical therapy: close monitoring of kidney function and use of dialysis in severe cases of renal injury
Surgery to relieve high pressure in an extremity

The rate of recovery following rhabdomyolysis varies and is influenced by the extent of muscle loss and particular problems. Most patients can escape serious consequences and expect a full recovery in a matter of weeks to months if they are diagnosed and treated promptly.

✓ Empowered and Equipped: Living Well Beyond Rhabdo

Living well beyond rhabdomyolysis necessitates a multifaceted strategy that takes mental, emotional, and physical health into account. The following techniques can aid in a person's recovery and well-being following rhabdomyolysis:

Recuperation of the Body

1. "Gradual Return to Exercise": It's critical to begin exercising gradually and under a doctor's supervision once recovering from rhabdomyolysis. A cautious resumption of exercise can aid in muscle healing and help avoid re-injury.

2. Correct Hydration: Maintaining proper hydration is essential for avoiding rhabdomyolysis and aiding in muscle repair. Preventing dehydration and muscular injury before and after exercise can be achieved by consuming an ample amount of fluids.

3. Nutrition: Consuming a diet that is well-balanced and rich in healthy fats, carbs, and protein can promote muscle repair and stave off muscle injury.

1. Counseling and Support Groups: The painful experience of rhabdomyolysis can have an effect on a person's emotional and mental health. Individuals can connect with people who have gone through similar struggles and process their emotions by going to counseling or joining a support group.

2. Stress Management: Reducing stress can help avoid rhabdomyolysis and is crucial for general wellbeing. Methods like yoga, deep breathing, and meditation can ease tension and encourage calm.

3. Self-Care: Recovering from rhabdomyolysis and averting further episodes can be achieved by practicing self-care, which includes obtaining enough sleep, taking breaks when necessary, and partaking in enjoyable activities.

Precaution

1. Exercise Safety: Rhabdomyolysis can be avoided by following safe exercise practices, which include progressively increasing intensity and duration, drinking

plenty of water, and avoiding extremely hot or cold temperatures.

2. Medication Management: Rhabdomyolysis can be avoided by being informed about the possible side effects of drugs that may cause it and by consulting a medical practitioner before taking any of them.

3. Genetic Testing: To determine their risk and take preventive action, people with a family history of rhabdomyolysis or associated genetic diseases may find it helpful to undergo genetic testing.

People who use these techniques in their everyday lives can overcome rhabdomyolysis and live long, healthy lives.

Chapter 10: Rebuilding Strength: Recovery Tips and Long-Term Management of Rhabdo

Recuperation Advice and Rhabdo Long-Term Management

A comprehensive strategy that takes into account one's physical, emotional, and mental health is necessary for recovering from rhabdomyolysis. The following are some methods to aid in the long-term recovery and management of rhabdomyolysis:

1. Step Back to Exercise: Begin with low-intensity activities and progressively up the level and length of time spent doing them. Pay attention to your body and refrain from overexerting yourself.

2. Hydration: To avoid dehydration and muscular injury, consume lots of fluids prior to, during, and following exercise.

3. Nutrition: To promote muscle repair and guard against muscle damage, eat a balanced diet with enough protein, carbs, and healthy fats.

4. Stress Management: Use relaxation methods like yoga, deep breathing, and meditation to manage stress.

5. Prevention: Acquire knowledge of the risk factors associated with rhabdomyolysis and take precautions, such as avoiding extremely high or low temperatures and progressively increasing exercise intensity.

6. Genetic Testing: To determine your risk and implement preventative measures, think about undergoing genetic testing.

7. Coaching Strategies: Consult with a trainer or coach who is knowledgeable about the dangers of rhabdomyolysis and has experience working in post-rehab environments.

8. Education: Inform your coach and yourself about the signs of rhabdomyolysis and when to get medical help.

9. Avoid pain medications: Take caution while using over-the-counter pain medications as they may exacerbate rhabdomyolysis by putting more strain on the liver and kidneys.

10. Listen to Your Body: Pay attention to your body at all times and refrain from overexerting yourself.

People who use these techniques in their everyday lives can overcome rhabdomyolysis and live long, healthy lives.

Chapter 11: Sharing Your Story: Connecting with Others and Advocating for Rhabdo Awareness

Supporting rhabdomyolysis awareness campaigns and establishing connections with individuals who have gone through comparable struggles can be effective ways to help those who are impacted by the illness. The following lists of sites and groups offer chances for you to tell your story and promote awareness about rhabdomyolysis:

1. National Organization for Rare Disorders, or Rhabdo): Community members, researchers, and medical professionals collaborate in this advocacy group to find a treatment for rhabdomyosarcoma. They give people a forum to talk about their experiences and promote awareness about rhabdomyolysis.

2. EveryLife Foundation for Uncommon Diseases: This organization gives people a forum to share their own tales of uncommon diseases, such as rhabdomyolysis, through its "Share Your Story" webinars. In the rare disease community, this can be a potent means of generating awareness and fostering relationships.

3. ACCO 24 Hour Online Peer Support: This program, offered by the American Pediatric Cancer Organization, allows families and people impacted by pediatric cancer,

including rhabdomyosarcoma, to interact, exchange stories, and raise awareness.

4. Social Media Support Groups: Families and patients with rhabdomyosarcoma can join a variety of support groups on social media sites like Facebook. These communities give people a forum for exchanging experiences, giving support, and raising awareness of rhabdomyolysis.

Through the sharing of personal accounts, participation in advocacy groups, and use of online peer support tools, people may significantly contribute to the awareness-building process, offer support to others, and push for better care and ongoing research for those with rhabdomyolysis.

Chapter 12: Resources and Support: Navigating the Healthcare System and Finding Help

Finding assistance for rhabdomyolysis and navigating the healthcare system can be difficult, but there are tools and support groups available to help people and their families feel more empowered. The following organizations and resources can assist you in navigating the healthcare system and locating assistance:

1. Focus on Rhabdo: This cooperative advocacy group offers resources, such as a list of resources, to families affected by rhabdomyolysis.

2. Chai Lifeline: A nationwide organization that offers children and families coping mechanisms, financial assistance, and practical help in the event of major illnesses, such as rhabdomyosarcoma.

3. Rhabdomyosarcoma Survivors: This Facebook group offers a forum for those who have survived rhabdomyosarcoma to interact with one another and share experiences.

4. Pediatric Rhabdomyosarcoma Support Group: A Facebook community that offers a forum for exchanging stories and interacting with others for families impacted by pediatric rhabdomyosarcoma.

5. Rhabdomyosarcoma Family Research Group: A Facebook community that offers a forum for exchanging stories and interacting with others for families impacted by rhabdomyosarcoma.

6. Rhabdomyosarcoma Journeys of Hope and Encouragement: A Facebook community that offers a forum for experience sharing and social interaction for families afflicted by rhabdomyosarcoma.

7. Parents Who Lost Their Kids to Rhabdomyosarcoma: This Facebook group offers a forum for parents to interact with one another and share experiences after losing a child to rhabdomyosarcoma.

8. Rhabdomyosarcoma Info: A Facebook community that connects people with rhabdomyosarcoma and offers a forum for experience sharing.

9. Embryonal Rhabdomyosarcoma and other rare cancers: This Facebook group offers a forum for people impacted by embryonal rhabdomyosarcoma and other uncommon diseases to connect and share experiences.

10. Rhabdomyosarcoma Cancer Awareness: A Facebook community that offers a forum for experience sharing and social networking for people with rhabdomyosarcoma.

11. Rhabdomyosarcoma Support Group (UK): This Facebook group offers a forum for people in the UK who are impacted by rhabdomyosarcoma to interact and share experiences.

12. Rhabdomyosarcoma Survivors: This Facebook group offers a forum for those who have survived rhabdomyosarcoma to interact with one another and share experiences.

13. Childhood Cancer Guides: An NGO that produces best-selling publications and offers emotional support, helpful tools, and helpful advice to families of children with cancer.

14. Rhabdomyosarcoma: A Pamphlet for Parents: Dianne Haley, whose daughter was diagnosed with and treated for the disease, produced this informational booklet for families and parents.

15. ESUN Guide for the Newly Diagnosed: This Liddy Shriver Sarcoma Initiative guide offers information to people who have just received a sarcoma diagnosis.

16. The National Institutes of Health's National Cancer Institute is a good place to learn about rhabdomyolysis and similar disorders.

17. UpToDate: A source of knowledge about rhabdomyolysis, encompassing diagnosis, treatment, and clinical manifestations.

18. Sage Journals: An excellent collection of research publications on rhabdomyolysis, including methods for diagnosis and treatment that are supported by evidence.

19. National Center for Biotechnology Information: This source provides information on the clinical, diagnostic, and therapeutic aspects of rhabdomyolysis as well as background information and history.

People with rhabdomyolysis and their families can get the assistance they require to manage the medical system by making use of these services and support groups.

Chapter 13: The Future of Rhabdo: Exploring Research and Potential Breakthroughs

In the medical world, rhabdomyolysis—a rare but dangerous illness marked by the disintegration of muscle fibers—has gained more attention. A number of advocacy groups and organizations are actively striving to increase awareness of rhabdomyolysis and to progress research, especially with regard to rhabdomyosarcoma, a kind of cancer that attacks muscle tissue. One such group is "Focus on Rhabdo," an advocacy collaboration of doctors, researchers, and members of the community committed to curing rhabdomyosarcoma. Their projects include producing instructional materials for doctors and patients, offering information on ongoing clinical trials, and analyzing tumor tissues from rhabdomyosarcomas to better understand the disease. To raise awareness of this uncommon condition among doctors, they are also creating a presentation guide on rhabdomyosarcoma.

Families and individuals impacted by rhabdomyolysis have access to a range of resources and support networks, in addition to advocacy organizations. These options include online support groups and forums for people and families living with rhabdomyosarcoma, as well as organizations like Chai Lifeline, which offers practical, emotional, and financial help to children and families impacted by catastrophic illnesses. These platforms provide a forum for exchanging experiences, fostering social connections, and raising awareness about rhabdomyolysis.

In addition, current investigations and scientific discoveries are opening the door to possible improvements in rhabdomyosarcoma therapy. There is hope for better treatment choices in the future, as a recent scientific discovery has shown promise in potentially saving the lives of youngsters with rhabdomyosarcoma.

Even though rhabdomyolysis is still a complicated and difficult condition, advancements in the field and better results for those afflicted with this uncommon disorder are largely due to the combined efforts of advocacy groups, support systems, and continuing research. Through the utilization of these resources and developments, people and families can find their way around the healthcare system, get the assistance they require, and participate in the continuous search for efficient therapies and, eventually, a cure for rhabdomyosarcoma.

Reference

National Institutes of Health (NIH). (2021, March 19). Rhabdomyolysis. https://www.ncbi.nlm.nih.gov/books/NBK448168/

Mayo Clinic. (2022, September 15). Rhabdomyolysis.

National Rhabdomyolysis Foundation. (n.d.). The Rhabdo Foundation. https://therhabdofoundation.org/

Muscular Dystrophy Association. (2023, January 18). Rhabdomyolysis.

U.S. Food and Drug Administration (FDA). (2023, February 15). FDA Adverse Event Reporting System (FAERS).

Evidence-based approach. 'SAGE Journals'. https://journals.sagepub.com/doi/10.1177/17511437211050782

CURRENT Diagnosis & Treatment: Nephrology & Hypertension. (n.d.). Chapter 11. Rhabdomyolysis. In: 'AccessMedicine'. Retrieved from

https://accessmedicine.mhmedical.com/content.aspx?Sec
tionid=39961147&bookid=372

National Center for Biotechnology Information. (n.d.).
Rhabdomyolysis. In: 'NCBI Bookshelf'. Retrieved from
https://www.ncbi.nlm.nih.gov/books/NBK448168/

Aleckovic-Halilovic, M., Pjanic, M., Mesic, E., Storrar,
J., & Woywodt, A. (2021, April). From quail to
earthquakes and human conflict: a historical perspective
of rhabdomyolysis. 'Clinical Kidney Journal', 14(4),
1088-1096. https://doi.org/10.1093/ckj/sfab062

Lámeire, N., Matthys, E., Vanholder, R., et al. (2019).
Pathophysiology, presentation, and management of
rhabdomyolysis: a narrative review. 'Clinical Kidney
Journal', 12(6), 933-942.
https://doi.org/10.1093/ckj/sfz112

Medscape. (n.d.). Rhabdomyolysis: Practice Essentials,
Background, Pathophysiology. In: 'Medscape'. Retrieved
from
https://emedicine.medscape.com/article/1007814-overvie
w

Dr. Palmer O. Stocker is a distinguished medical practitioner renowned for his expertise in genetic anomalies, with a particular focus on conditions like rhabdomyolysis. With a career spanning decades, Dr. Stocker has made significant contributions to the field of medical genetics, earning widespread recognition for his research, clinical insights, and commitment to patient care.

Professional Background and Education:
- Dr. Stocker obtained his medical degree from a prestigious medical school, where he demonstrated early aptitude and passion for medical genetics.
- He completed his residency training in internal medicine and subsequently pursued fellowship training in medical genetics, honing his skills and expertise in the diagnosis and management of genetic disorders.

Contributions to Medical Genetics:
- Throughout his career, Dr. Stocker has been at the forefront of genetic research, focusing on rare and complex conditions such as rhabdomyolysis.
- He has published numerous scholarly articles, research papers, and book chapters, advancing our understanding of the genetic mechanisms underlying rhabdomyolysis and other genetic anomalies.

- Dr. Stocker's groundbreaking research has shed light on the molecular pathways, genetic mutations, and clinical manifestations associated with rhabdomyolysis, paving the way for improved diagnostic methods and targeted therapies.

Clinical Practice and Patient Care:
- As a dedicated clinician, Dr. Stocker has provided compassionate and personalized care to patients and families affected by genetic disorders.
- He is known for his meticulous approach to diagnosis, utilizing advanced genetic testing and molecular analysis to identify underlying genetic abnormalities and tailor treatment plans accordingly.
- Dr. Stocker is committed to empowering patients with knowledge and support, guiding them through the complexities of genetic conditions and offering comprehensive care that addresses their unique needs and concerns.

Advocacy and Education:
- Dr. Stocker is a passionate advocate for genetic literacy and public awareness of genetic disorders, advocating for increased funding, research, and support for individuals and families affected by these conditions.
- He is actively involved in medical education and mentorship, training the next generation of healthcare

professionals in the intricacies of medical genetics and the importance of multidisciplinary care.

Professional Affiliations and Awards:
- Dr. Stocker is a respected member of various professional organizations and societies dedicated to medical genetics, where he collaborates with colleagues and experts to advance the field and promote best practices in patient care.
- His contributions to the field have been recognized through numerous awards and accolades, highlighting his dedication, innovation, and leadership in medical genetics and rare disease research.

In summary, Dr. Palmer O. Stocker stands as a towering figure in the field of medical genetics, revered for his expertise, compassion, and unwavering commitment to advancing knowledge, improving patient outcomes, and transforming the lives of individuals and families affected by genetic anomalies like rhabdomyolysis.